The Magic of Mustard

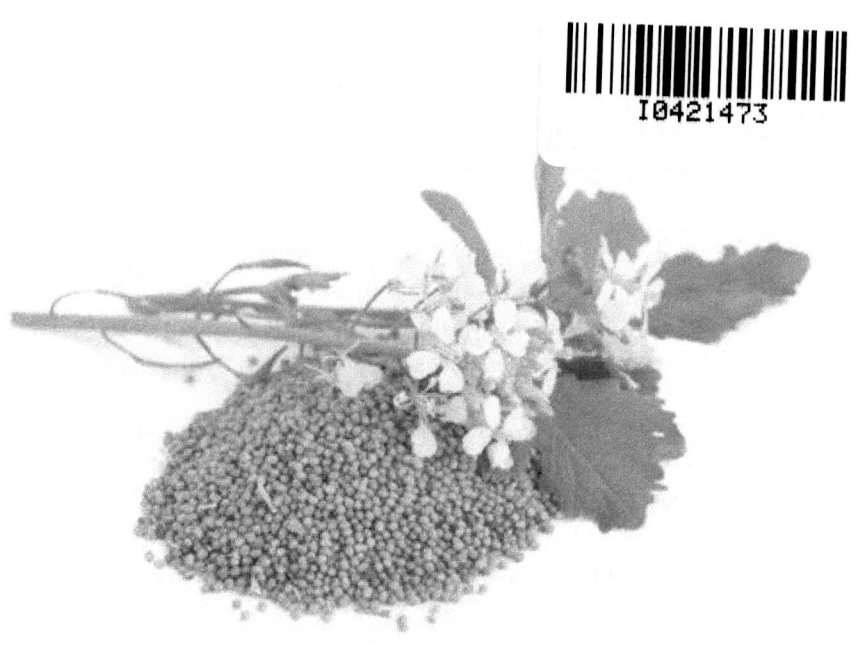

Healthy Learning Series

Dueep Jyot Singh

Mendon Cottage Books

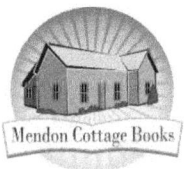

JD-Biz Publishing

Disclaimer

The information is this book is provided for informational purposes only. It is not intended to be used and medical advice or a substitute for proper medical treatment by a qualified health care provider. The information is believed to be accurate as presented based on research by the author.

The contents have not been evaluated by the U.S. Food and Drug Administration or any other Government or Health Organization and the contents in this book are not to be used to treat cure or prevent disease.

The author or publisher is not responsible for the use or safety of any diet, procedure or treatment mentioned in this book. The author or publisher is not responsible for errors or omissions that may exist.

Warning

The Book is for informational purposes only and before taking on any diet, treatment or medical procedure, it is recommended to consult with your primary health care provider.

Our books are available at

1. Amazon.com

2. Barnes and Noble

3. Itunes

4. Kobo

5. Smashwords

6. Google Play Books

Table of Contents

Introduction

The moment you hear the word "he is as keen as mustard", you immediately visualize a person bubbling over with enthusiasm. The word mustard in itself brings on an idea of a pungent and delicious condiment, without which you may not enjoy your hamburgers, meat steaks, and other preparations. We *just* need that extra touch of mustard to add to the flavor of an otherwise bland dish.

The old Romans knew all about it when they prepared a mixture of young wine –mustum-and mustard seeds and ground them together into a paste. The ard portion of the word comes from the Latin word for hot and flaming –ardens, as in ardent...

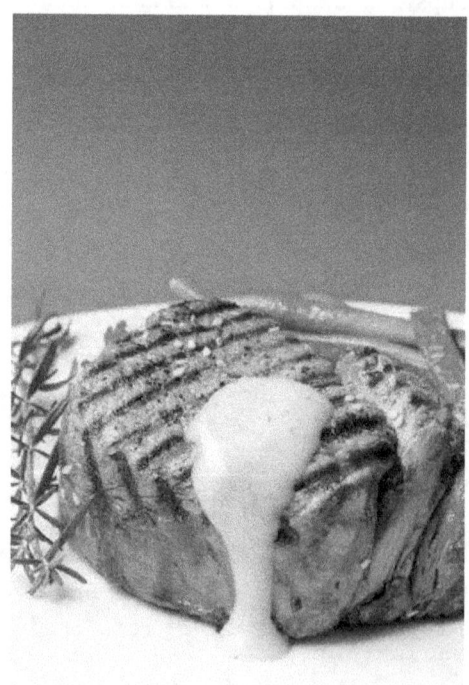

An ancient Roman recipe book, which was found in the fourth century spoke about a mustard sauce, which was made up of a mixture of grilled coriander seeds, pepper, ground mustard, Bishops weed, Caraway, onion, thyme, celery, oregano, honey, oil, lovage, fish sauce, and vinegar.

This was then used as a glaze for roasting boar, especially on the pit. Those Romans did not seem to have forgotten anything in the herbs and spices list.

But then mustard was a spice, which has been known for millenniums and has been part and parcel of mankind's culinary expertise. When the Romans conquered Gaul, they took mustard along with them, and by the 10th century, French monks had learned all the ancient secrets of growing and preparing mustard. By the 12th century, Dijon mustard was famous throughout Europe.

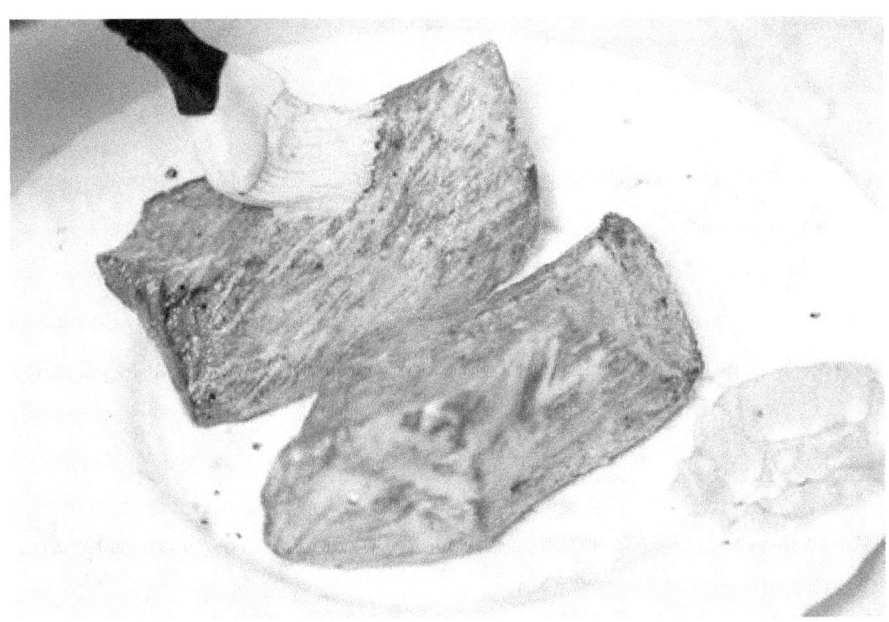

Imagine the quantities of mustard being eaten by the French, as shown in an ancient French history book. The Duke of Burgundy, invited his nobles and families to a grand gala somewhere in 1396. They managed to finish *70 gallons* of a preparation known as mustard crème! Talk about digestive powers!

Hot dogs without mustard is unimaginable, but these hot dogs were eaten without mustard until 1904, when they were tested out by the RT company at the world's fair held in St. Louis. And since then, it is "Where Is the Mustard with My Hamburgers and Hotdogs"?[1]

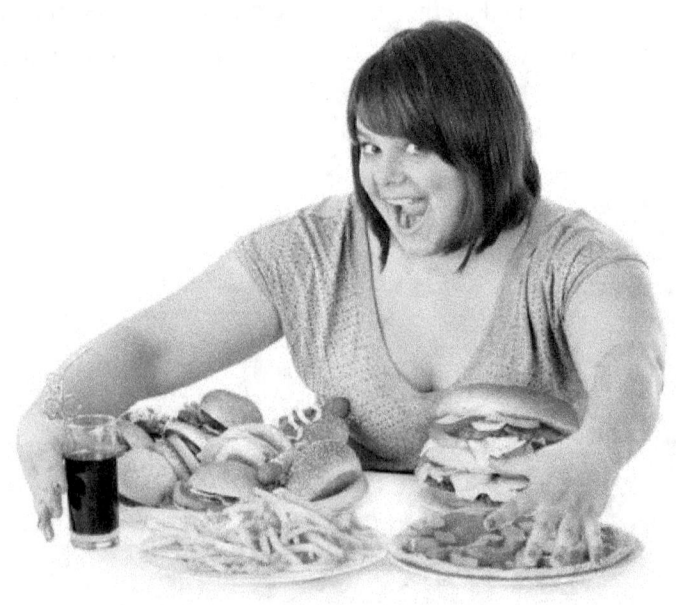

---

[1] I do that, even at my advanced age, – especially when I am eating greasy hotdogs, and even sausages and bacon – and of course, they have to be accompanied with tomato ketchup in huge quantities. Also mustard with cold meat and horseradish is a must. No fun if any of these ingredients are missing when you are eating cold meat.

Now this is about the popularity of the mustard in the West. What about the East? In excavations going back more than 4000 BC in the Indus Valley, and other parts of Asia, mustard seeds have been found as part of the crops grown by the farmers.

In the holy Bible, the mustard seed has been compared to God's kingdom, which grows and flourishes from a small seed. Just one small seed can grow up into such a huge and beneficial plant.

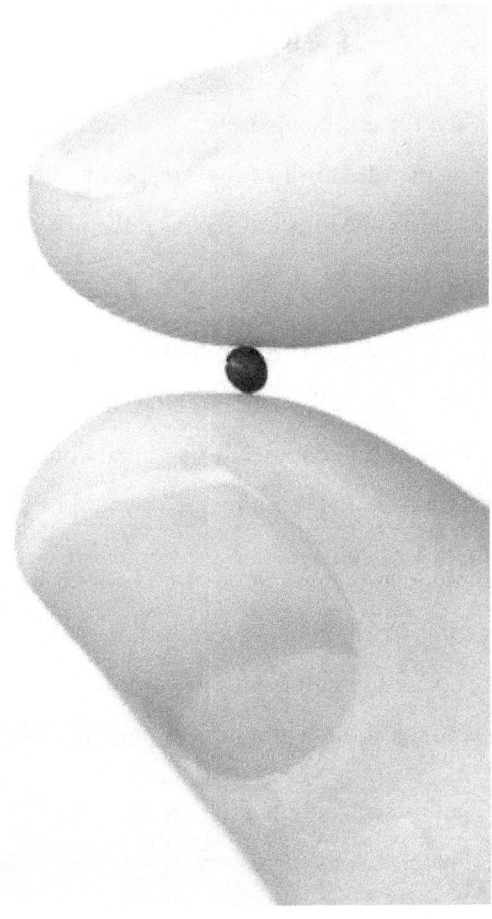

A Biblical symbol of Faith...

In ancient Buddhist mythology, a grieving widow who had lost her only son came to the Buddha and requested him to revive him. The Lord told her to go around the country and get a handful of mustard seeds from any house where death had not set foot. She soon found out that death was universal and reconciled herself to his loss.

Here is another interesting traditional story I heard as a child. I was bemoaning the fact that my face and body was sprinkled with tiny black moles. My grandmother told me that I must have been a good soul, doing a lot of good deeds or a rich and prosperous person in my last reincarnation!

That is why when I was cremated, the whole city arrived there with handfuls of mustard seeds in order to show their respect and regard for the late lamented. They threw the mustard seeds on the body, which was then cremated.

According to her, my skin like any newborn's was unblemished when I was born, but as I grew, nature brought out those moles on the skin surface in order to remind me to do good deeds like I had done in the past! So that when I left this time around mustard seeds would be thrown on my body in farewell, before it was consigned to the flames.

I have not seen this tradition being followed in the 21st century, but it was a part of Eastern social life in the days of yore. But what an excellent way of keeping people to the straight and narrow, and the path of Good!

The mustard plant is such an integral part of Eastern culture, that one of the top Bollywood blockbusters of yesteryear had the hero and heroine meeting each other after a long separation in a field of fresh yellow mustard, blooming away in the spring.[2] Since then, dancing in the mustard field, in the spring either with your partner or with other hep youngsters of the village/city has become one of the old and timeworn film clichés in Bollywood.

---

[2] This Movie has run continuously for 20 years, in some theaters. https://www.youtube.com/watch?v=c25GKI5VNeY – enjoy the trailer.

The movie title literally means – The Brave Hearts Will Take Away the Bride – somewhat on the Only the Brave Deserve the Fair theme.

Varieties

The common white mustard – *Brassica juncea* – is a native to the Mediterranean region, North Africa, and other parts of the East, from where it was taken by traders and travelers to the rest of the world. This is largely grown for salads, and greens, and slowly began to be replaced with spinach and kale in the 20th century.

Oriental White Mustard is a native to the Himalayas and is grown commercially in Denmark, Canada, India, as well as the US. This plant is a hardy annual of the Cruciferae family.

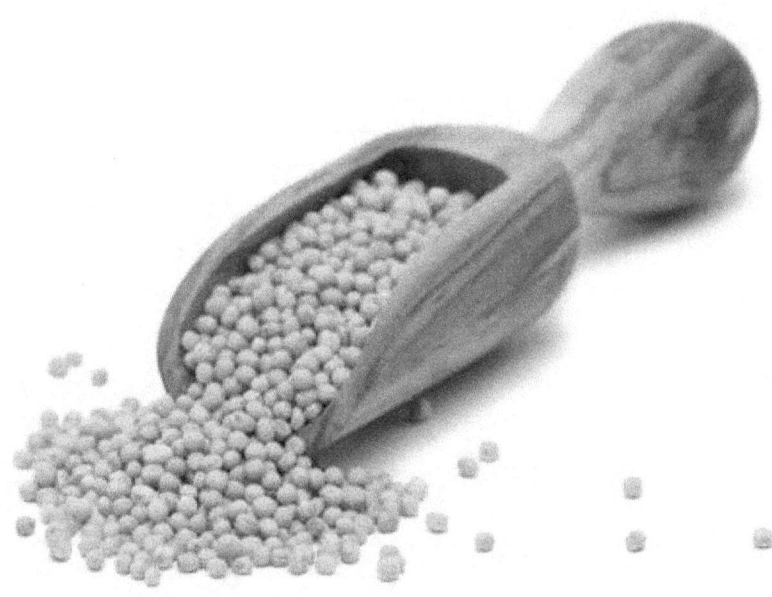

Brassica nigra, or the black mustard is grown extensively for its seed, which is made into the mustard of commerce. It is grown in the US, Chile, Argentina, and of course, this is the mustard, which you enjoy as a condiment preparation, especially when it comes from the UK or from France. Nepal and Canada together produce 57% of the world's mustard production.

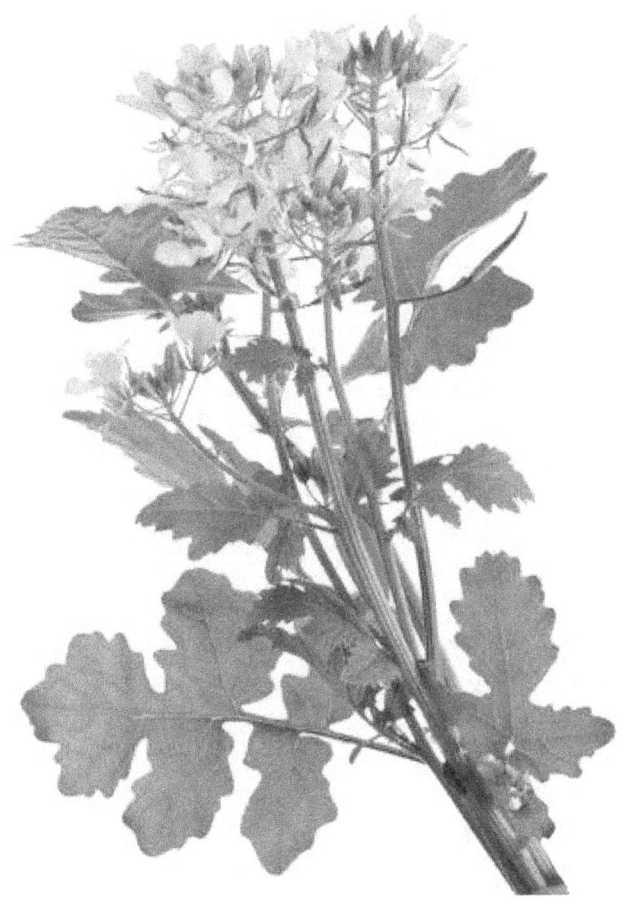

Brassica campestris or brown mustard is very popular in the Indian sub-continent with the leaves cooked as a staple food and eaten extensively in the winter. The yellow mustard is also a variety of *Brassica campestris, variety sarson.*

The Chinese Pak Choi variety grows in 60 days and Bok Choi (yes, they are different varieties with similar sounding names – grows in 45 days.) So does Joi Choi, and the broadleaved Florida variety. Dai gai and Choi Sum take 60 days to get ready for harvest.

Cultivation

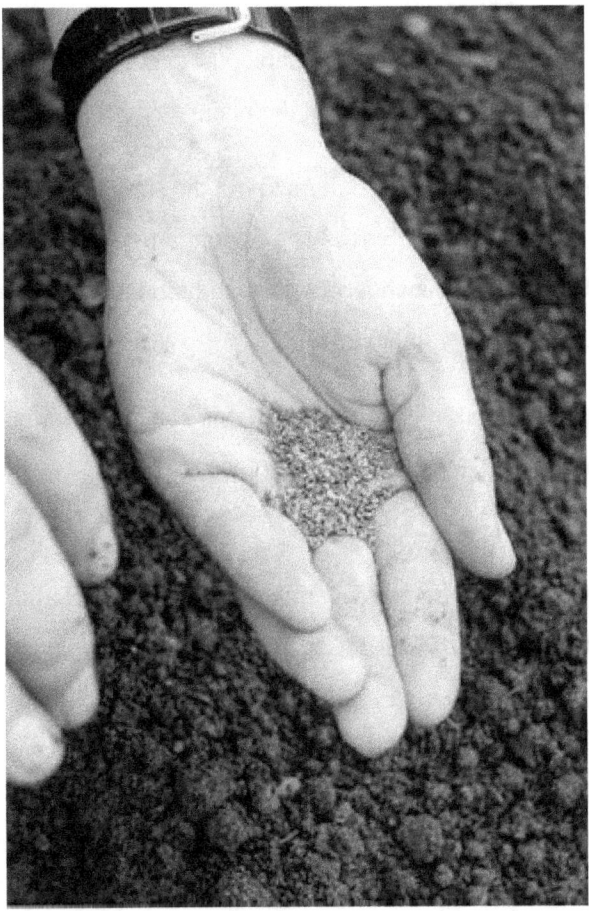

Mustard seeds are small and round, with their colors ranging from yellowish white to brown and black. They are tiny, just about two millimeters in diameter.

The mustard seed is sown very early in the spring for spring use. It is also sown in the fall for a winter crop. The seeds are sown from the middle of September to the end of November, especially in the plains . If you are planning mustard in the years, sewing is going to be carried out during May to July. For raising mustard as a vegetable, the seeds are sown at about 35 cm apart in rows than 10 cm between the plants.

 The plants are going to go to seed quickly in the spring. You can thin out the plants as they crowd in the row. The thinning distance can be anywhere between four inches to 12 inches apart, depending on how much space you have, and which variety you have sown.

For the larger leafed varieties, you need higher spacing where the seed is sown thickly in drills 13 – 15 inches apart.

In ancient times, the seeds were broadcast by hand, because they were so tiny that farmers did not bother covering them up with soil after sowing, as they would do for normal plant seeds. 10 kg of seeds were necessary for broadcasting in 1 hectare of prepared land. But if you are planting by hand, you may want to have around eight kilograms per hectare because you may not be quite certain about the germination rate of the plants.

This is because mustard seeds have a number of natural enemies, which are just waiting for them to be planted. These include insects and rats. So I would suggest starting up seedlings in a pot, and then planting them by hand later on.

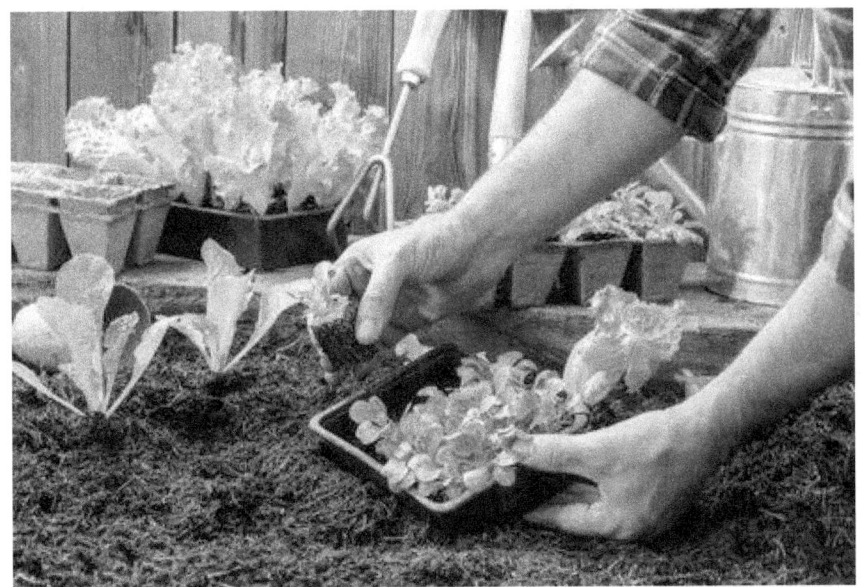

Vegetable seedlings either planted outdoors after they have been bought in a nursery, or those seedlings started right at home in potting compost

Make sure that the seed that is prepared beforehand with plenty of fertilizer to get good results. Soil which is rich in humus is going to give you extremely good crops. The best soil for a mustard crop is a good sandy loamy soil. It should also be rich in nitrogen, phosphorus, and potash.

Brassica japonica has two varieties – *The Ostrich Plume* and *The Giant Curled.* These have large leaves.

Growth and Harvest

The seeds are going to take anywhere between 5 – 10 days for germination, depending on the weather. The climate and the soil requirements are just the same to that of any other winter leafy vegetable – i.e. if you are living in an area where there is no killer frost around, you are going to enjoy mustard throughout the winter.

The average temperature should be around 75 degrees Fahrenheit. As this is a leafy vegetable, which is a cool season crop you can so the mustard seeds, as early as four – six weeks before the possible last and average frost date in the spring.

Farmers normally rotate this mustard crop, every 4 – 6 weeks so that it can produce crops every 30 – 40 days to give you a rich harvest.

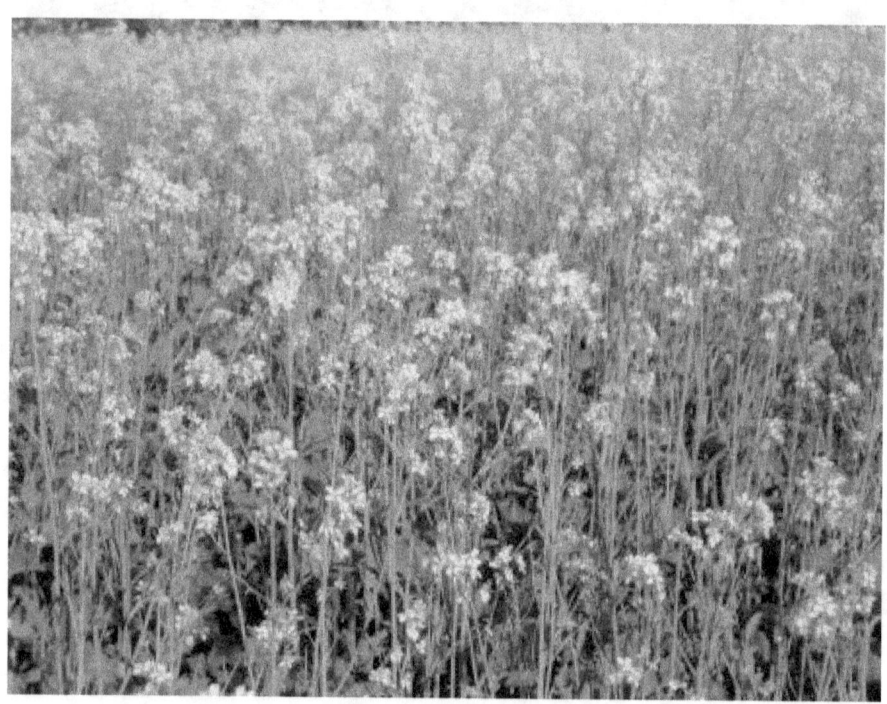

If you are living in a region where the winter is mild, you can sow the mustard in the early winter or in the autumn itself.

If you are growing mustard for your family, 6 – 10 plants of mustard for each family member is going to serve you well. The best peppery flavor of the stem as well as the leaves is best obtained 25 – 30 days after you sow it.

Mustard plants love the full sun or partial shade. Harvesting is normally done by removing the leaves you want, and if you want the optimal result of seeds, you are going to leave a large amount of leaves on the plant itself, during the harvesting.

The soil pH value should be anywhere between 5.5 – 6.5. If the soil is colder than 40 degrees Fahrenheit, you may find the seeds reluctant to germinate.

If you grow mustard in the summer, you are going to get just seeds. You can consider these plants to have "bolted."

Mustard needs plenty of moisture in the soil, in order to grow quickly. The soil is never kept dry. You can prepare the soil beforehand by adding compost to the bed and allowing the compost to disintegrate for about one or two months, before you decide to do the sowing. In the midseason, you can add a layer of compost to the soil, to nourish the growing plants.

Continuous de-weeding is necessary. Mustard is a self-seeding plant, so you have to make sure that the mustard harvest is done before the plant goes into seed. Otherwise, next year you are going to find your land overflowing with mustard plants.

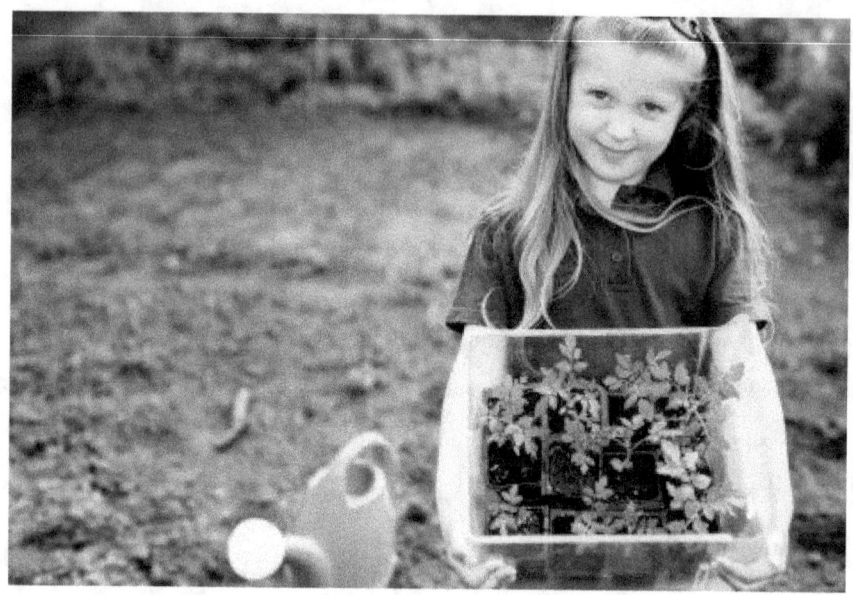

Seedlings of any plant have a better chance of survival outdoors, than seeds sown freshly.

Container growing of mustard is a good idea. Just broadcast the seed in your container filled with good potting medium and sprinkle the topmost layer lightly with soil.

Pests like aphids can be kept away by sprinkling the leaves with water. Make sure the water does not remain on the leaves, because then it is going to cause white rust, which is a fungus caused due to excess of moisture. Watering is always done at the base of the stem and soil, so that the leaves do not get wet.

Harvesting is done when the leaves are about two – three inches long. You can also use the entire plant after you have cut it. The harvesting is done before the summer sets in, because if the plants are allowed to grow in the summer, you are going to have really strong tasting leaves which are tough.

Storage

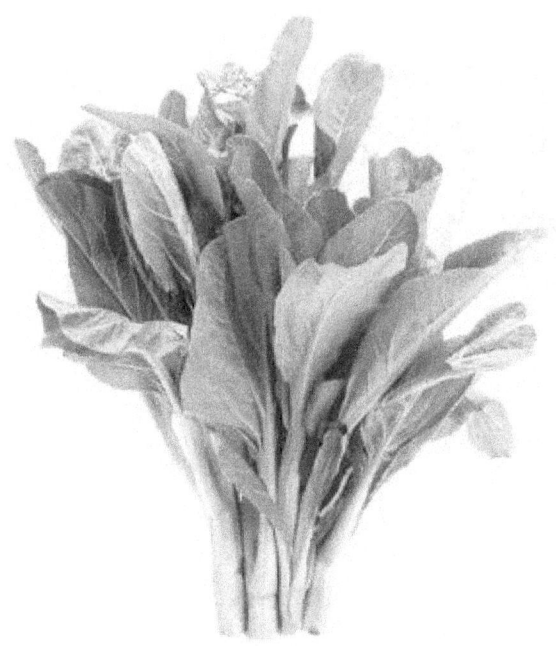

Storage of mustard leaves can be done in your fridge's vegetable compartment for anywhere between 1 to 2 weeks, if you wrap it up in a natural cloth bag, which is absorbent. At room temperature, it is going to start turning yellow and unless you want dried mustard, you may want to eat the green leaves right now as a salad or as a vegetable.

Mustard Seed Oil

Mustard is an invaluable producer of mustard seed oil, which is not only used extensively all over the world are cooking, but it is also used since ancient times for healing purposes.

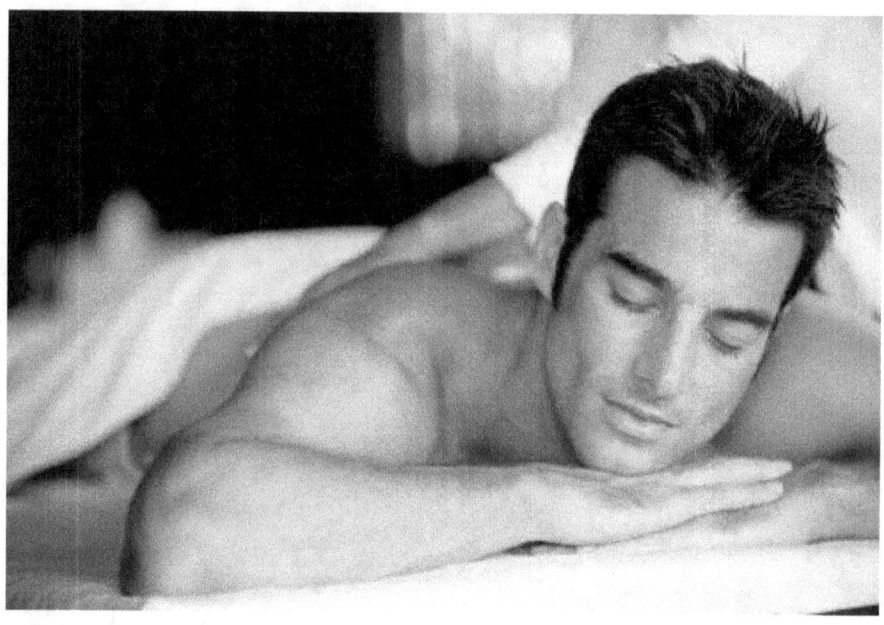

Even now mustard seed is used in many parts of the world in order to massage the skin, to keep it healthy, glowing, and disease-free. Mustard oil is also used in many parts of Asia as a hair oil in order to get well-managed, long growing dark tresses.

This oil is very pungent in smell and it is very strong. That is why it is applied to the skin directly, in very small quantities. Black and brown mustard seeds are going to give you larger quantities of oil when compared with the yellow varieties.

The world's major producers of mustard seed apart from Canada and Nepal, which produces 57 percent of the world's mustard produce are Hungary, the United States, countries in the Indian subcontinent and Great Britain.

When my father was a youngster, he used to speak about daily massages given to him by his grandmother in order to make him strong and sturdy. The massage oil was a mixture of mustard oil and Taramira oil, the latter of which I had never heard the name. It is an oil extracted from Eruca sativa seeds. It is stronger than mustard and pungent.

This particular plant is grown extensively in West Asia, where it is used as a cooking medium, as a salad oil, and also for pickling.

Mustard seed cake has been used as a very important fertilizer for millenniums. The seed cake is also used to feed cattle in many Asian countries. You can also use this seed cake as an excellent natural pesticide.

Mustard oil is very proteinaceous and that is why you may find yourself eating dishes with the flavor of mustard, if you enjoy West Asian cuisine.

This oil is considered to be The Oil in which to fry pieces of fish in many parts of these, just like it is considered to be the necessary accompaniment for cold meat dishes in the West.

If you are not bothered about the neighbors complaining of the strong smell of frying fish, you may want to try it out at least once. Remember to have the mustard oil smoking hot in the Wok. It is going to turn white instead of pale yellow – brown. "Uncooked" mustard oil is going to spoil the taste of your fish.

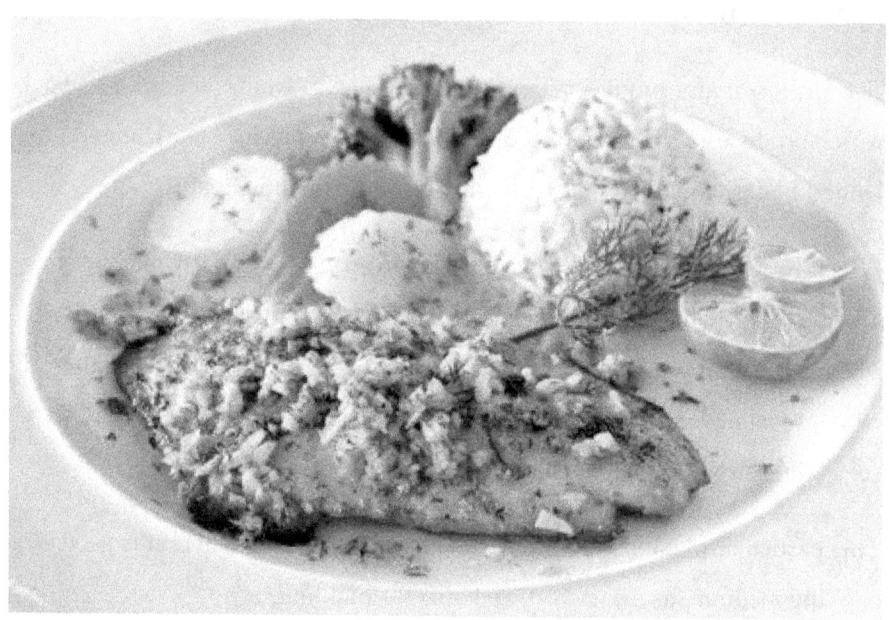

Put the filets of the fish in the oil, when it has finished smoking, and you have switched off the fire. This oil is now going to instill the mustard flavor in the fish. Fry the fish, as you would do it in any other oil and drain before serving. Sprinkle leaves of parsley before serving.

Culinary Uses of Mustard

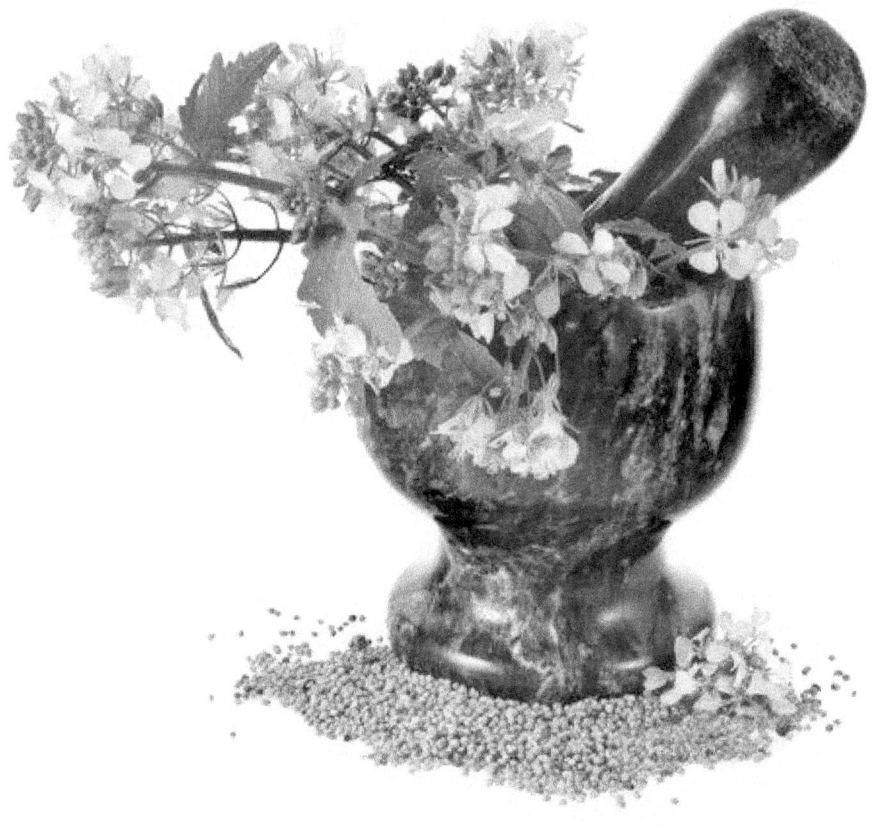

So, well, Apicius in ancient Rome, could not do without his mustard sauce all over his roast boar. Some sort of Mustard seed sauce made up with wine, lemon juice, vinegar, water and salt or any other liquids is going to be found in any cuisine on the earth of which you could think.

It is going to be made into a paste, along with herbs, spices and flavorings. It is going to be spicy, sweet and sour or just its own pungent flavor. The color of the sauces can range anywhere between golden yellow to brownish-black.

You can use it liberally with cheese and meat products, stakes, sandwiches, hamburgers, and tofu. You can also use it in salad dressings, soups, glazes, marinades and sauces.

In many parts of Asia, and in the Mediterranean region, as well as in Africa, South Eastern Europe and the Americas, you are going to find mustard, either in its seed form, or in its sauce form being used in the cuisine to add piquancy to dishes and make them more palatable.

Is it a wonder that mustard is one of the most extensively used and best loved of condiments in the world.

Brands

So when you ask for hot mustard from a seller, what do you expect? A mixture of brown or black mustard seeds mixed up with any sort of cold liquid to bring out the pungency and piquancy. You can also take your choice from these world-famous brands – Grey Poupon, Düsseldorfer Löwensenf, Maille, Colman's Heinz and French's [remember the "'s" mark, in the latter named brand.]

You may also want to try the Asian variety, which is known as Kasundi. It is strong and is used extensively, in regular meals, as an accompaniment for street food and fruit salads, or just as a sandwich paste.

The homemade mayonnaise recipe made every three weeks in our kitchen does not use English mustard or Dijon. It uses Kasundi because we like our mayonnaise, strong and pungent with lots of garlic in it, giving it a Provencal or Italian flavor.

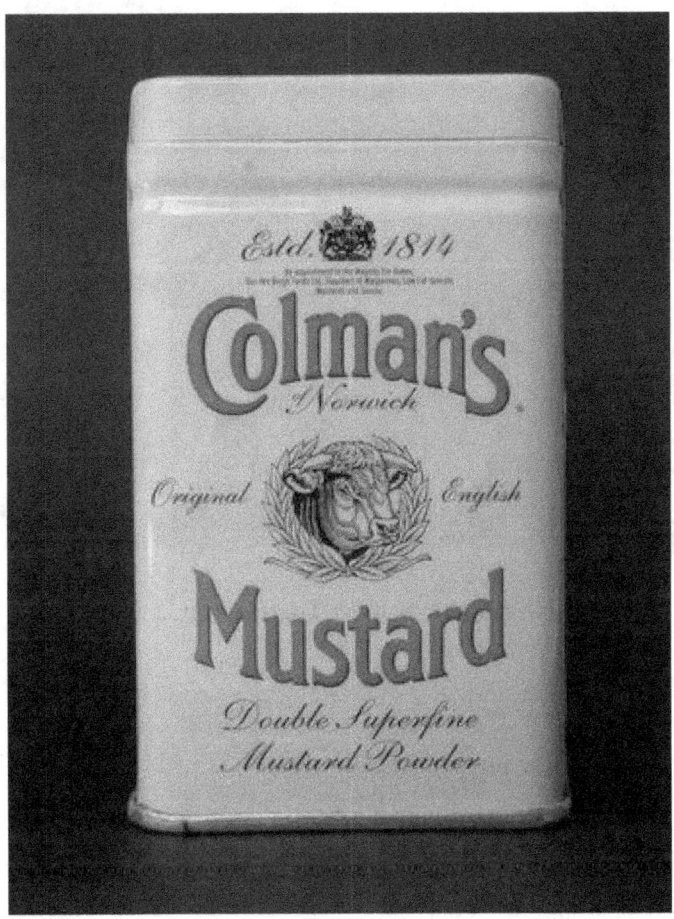

Remember that any preparation which you make of mustard at home is going to be hotter. It is also going to have a more intense flavor than the preparations you buy commercially. So be careful about the amount of mustard you add to your original mustard preparation recipe.

Pickles and Preserving

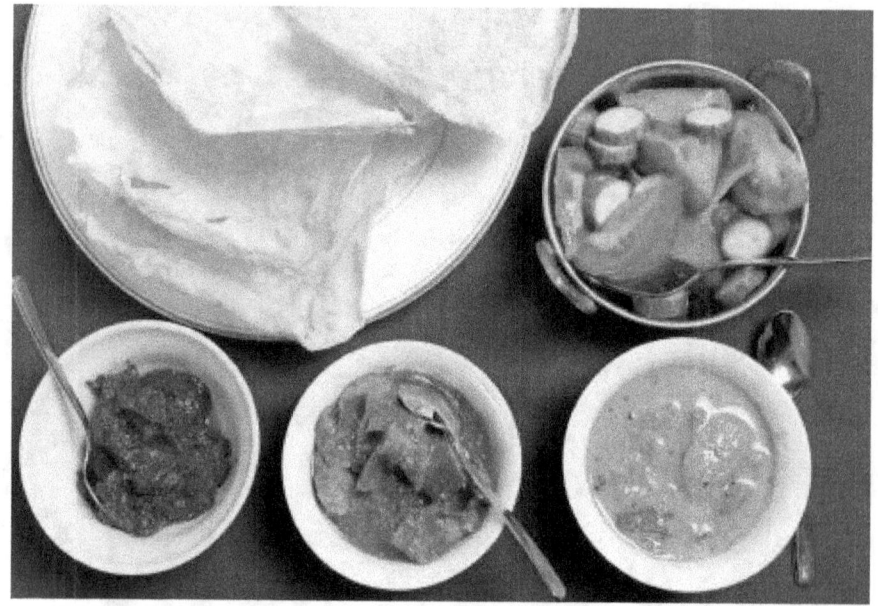

Pickles, condiments, King Tastemaker... Mustard.

I remember as a child, a neighbor getting ready to pickle the season's left over harvest of vegetables. She had lots of mustard oil at hand. She also made sure that she had about two handfuls of brown mustard seeds, along with other spices and dried herbs.

She used to fry the spices and salt in smoking hot mustard oil, before she added the vegetables to the spice mixture.

When the vegetables were cooked, they were placed in a glass jar, and more mustard oil poured on them. They were then allowed to cook in the sun throughout the summer.

These pickles used to last anywhere between 3 to 5 years, because ever so often, she would add cooked mustard oil to the vegetables in order to preserve them. This traditional way of making pickles has been handed down the generations for millenniums.

Sauces and Soups

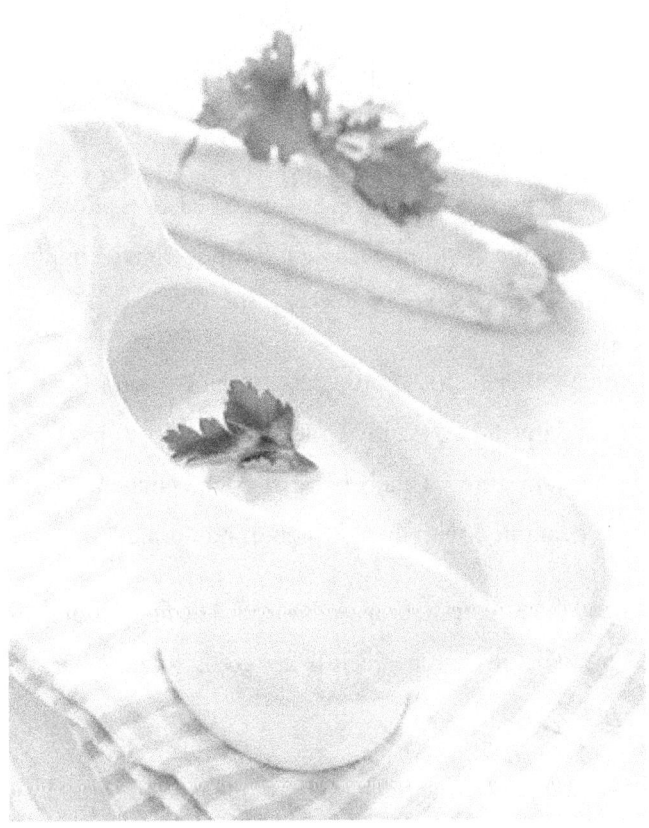

Hollandaise sauce without mustard? I think not!

I once enjoyed a delicious mustard soup in the house of a Belgian friend. When I asked her for the recipe, she said "guess." So all of us at the party began to guess what was in the soup. When I said mustard, she said, "how do you know?" I recognized that particular taste, having been brought up on it. Other ingredients in the soup were chopped bacon, plenty of cream, garlic and parsley.

She also told me another secret of making the perfect sauce Hollandaise. One teaspoonful of mustard is going to prevent the sauce from curdling.

Dry mustard in itself is not going to show its magic; you need to add water or any other liquid in order to get the full power and flavor out of the bruised seeds.

Mustard loses its pungency when it is heated. So always add it afterwards, after you have done the cooking, instead of while you are cooking. One teaspoonful of mustard is going to give you five calories.

Let me tell you another secret of prepared mustard – hotter liquids are going to give you a mild mustard mixture. Colder liquids are going to give you really hot mustard mixtures. This is because of the pungency producing enzymes being denatured with the addition of hot liquids.

You do not need to refrigerate prepared mustard because it has powerful antibacterial properties. That means it is not going to grow harmful bacteria, mildew or fungi.

Once you have prepared some mustard, by crushing the seeds in wine or vinegar – temperature according to the requirement of the strength of the mustard needed – place it in the refrigerator so that you do not need to worry about loss of strength as time goes by.

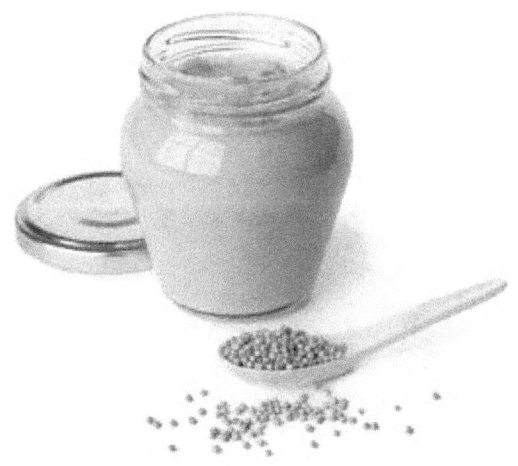

You may find some of this prepared mustard separated from the liquid in which it has been mixed. This happens if you have not use the mustard for a long time. Just give it a stir, and you are going to have a powerful mixture again.

Mustard is going to turn bitter, if you leave unrefrigerated for a long time. That is the reason why, in olden times when there were no refrigerators around people used to store their mustard preparations in cold cellars.

Dijon , being the mustard capital of the world is going to give you a medium strength preparation. Stronger mustards can be obtained in Düsseldorf and Norwich.

These preparations are going to vary on the amounts of herbs and spices added during the preparation process.

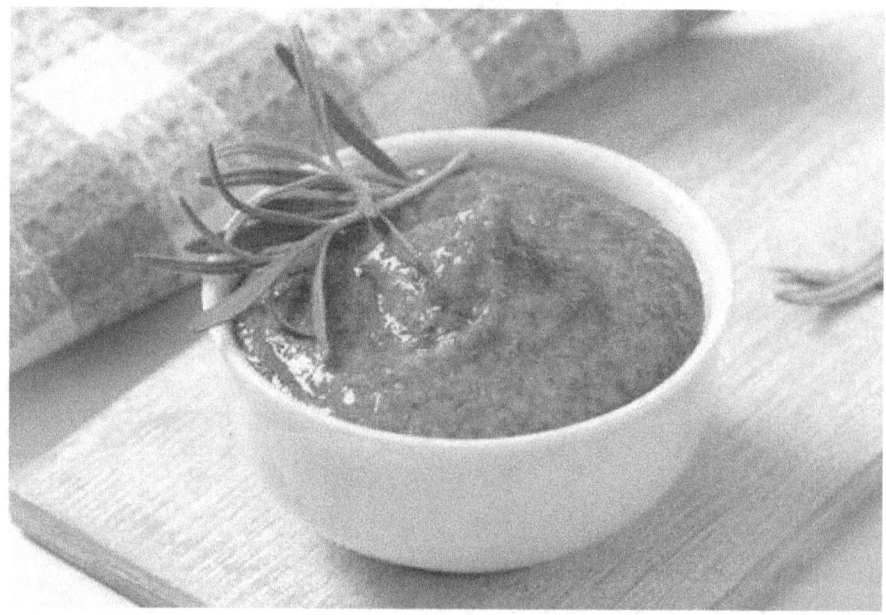

In Bavaria, the mustard which is prepared is sweet, because lots of sugar is added for preservation purposes instead of salt and herbs.

In Ireland, where we cannot do without the Water of Life, mustard is always going to be prepared with the addition of whiskey. What an interesting use of whiskey.

Preparing Mustard at Home

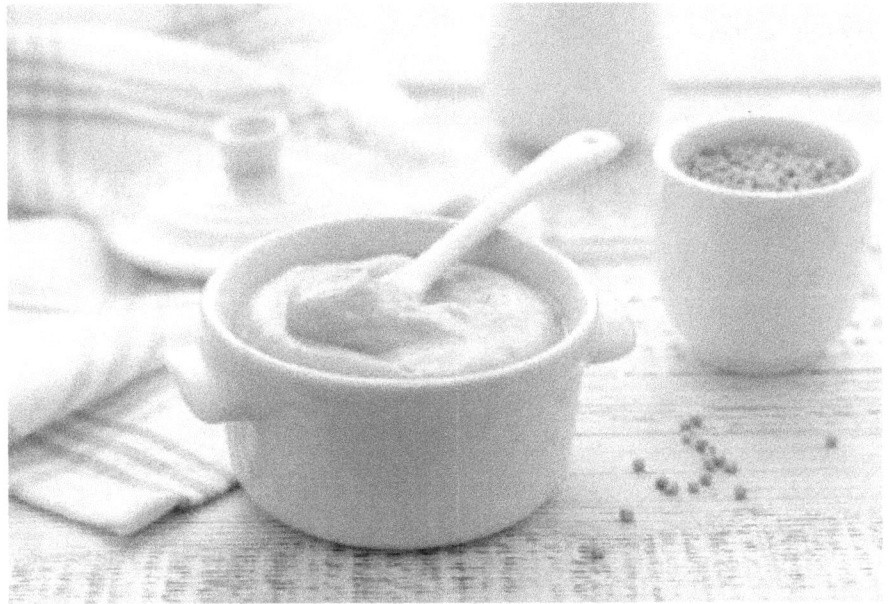

This is the traditional way in which you are going to prepare mustard at home, especially if you are in the habit of buying it off the shelf in large quantities.

You may want to do your own experimentation by taking wheat flour, mustard seed, herbs and spices and turmeric in enough of quantities to make a smooth paste. I would suggest 1/8 of a teaspoonful of turmeric. Now you can add beer, vinegar and wine and allow this mixture to stand for about 10 minutes before serving with meat.

You are going to prepare it before you dish up the meal. I am using the other liquids, because if you prepare it with water, it is going to be strong, but it is going to just deteriorate if you get a little late in serving it.

Try this recipe –

http://honest-food.net/2010/10/18/how-to-make-mustard/

I normally use honey or one tablespoonful of Canadian maple syrup, just for the Zing Thing.

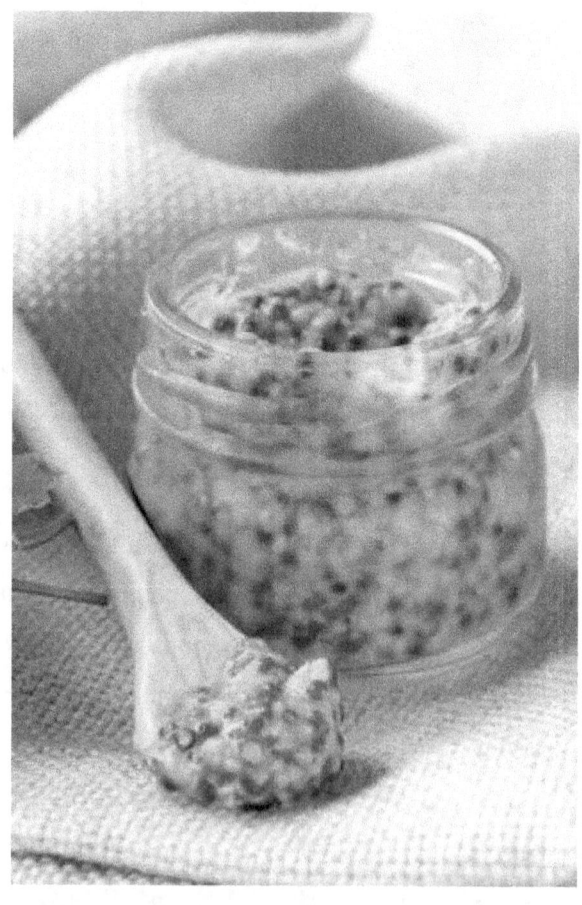

The yellow mustard which you grab off the supermarket shelves is dark yellow in color. That is because turmeric has been added to it. In many parts of Europe, beer is substituted for vinegar, so you may find beer-based mustard served up to you somewhere if you are a globetrotter.

The world-famous Dijon mustard was created just by mere chance, when M.Naigeon, a Dijon mustard maker, not having any vinegar around substituted unripe grape juice in his mustard preparation and wowed the world. Nowadays, this mustard is more prone to have wine in it, instead of grape juice.

Colman's English mustard is famous for its thick consistency, and hot, pungent flavor. This of course is made of English mustard yellow colored seeds and has been a popular condiment since 1814.

Just imagine that you are walking down the supermarket aisles. You are confronted with French mustard. Aha , you say, the real French stuff. But no, you look at the labels carefully. It says French mustard made by Colman. This was made in 1936, for all those people who did not like really strong mustard with their meat for lunch.

You may find it rarely on the shelves now, because production of this particular brand was stopped in 2001, but people still continue manufacturing this milder version locally. Along with this, you can find Honey mustard combinations mixed with olive oil and vinegar to be used as salad dressings and dips or for grilled meat baste.

Traditional French Mayonnaise

You are going to get about 1.5 cups (340 mL) of this traditional mayonnaise with the ingredients given. This is supposed to have been invented somewhere around 1756, in Minorca. The word comes from moyeun- [egg yolks]-aise-mixture/ sauce. It would also have been derived from the word *manier* , which means to stir up and is the corrupted pronunciation of *magnonaise* – or stirred up mixture.

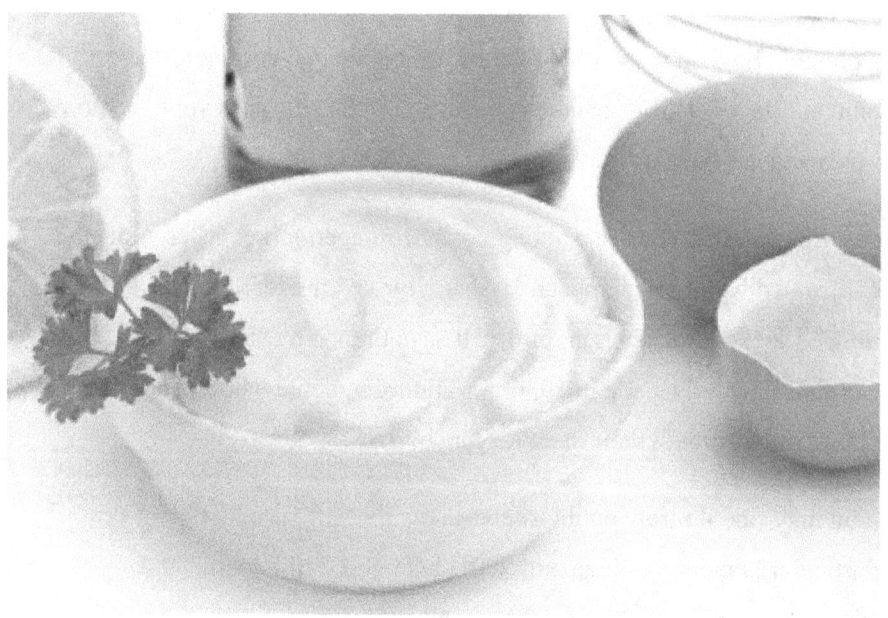

<u>**French Mayonnaise**</u>

- **Two egg yolks**

- **Two Tbsp of lemon juice or wine vinegar**

- **Half a tsp of prepared mustard**

- One pinch of salt

- One pinch of white pepper

- About 1 1/2 cups (350 mL) of olive oil or a combination of sunflower and olive oil

- One Tbsp of boiling water

Traditionally, this is beaten by the hand. Place the egg yolks in a mixing bowl with a few drops of vinegar. Add the white pepper and salt to taste. Started beating slowly with a wire whisk, adding the oil drop by drop. You are going to emulsify the egg yolks.

Beat this consistently. When the mixture is very thick, you can thin it with a few drops of vinegar. You can also add the rest of the ingredients as you want, while beating. Once the oil has been used up, gradually beat in the boiling water.

This is going to improve the consistency and help in the prevention of separation of the ingredients. Once a mayonnaise has been made, bottle it in a glass jar and either store in a cool, dry place, or in the refrigerator.

Aïoli – Traditional Butter of Provence

This is going to make about 6 ounces (170 mL). This is normally called the butter of Provence and is very popular in this particular area, as well as the Nice area. This is a thick, spicy, and garlicky mayonnaise. You are going to serve it as a dip for potatoes, green beans, cooked vegetables, and raw vegetables- crudités- [croo- dee tay-].

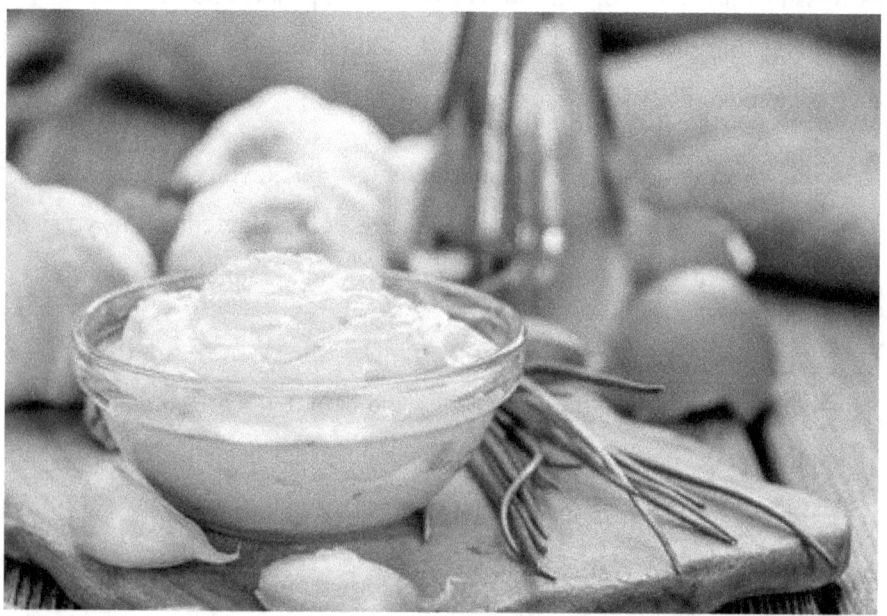

Aïoli

- 8 crushed garlic cloves

- One egg yolk (at room temperature)

- Cayenne pepper & salt to taste

- **1/8 tsp of prepared vinegar**

- **About 6 ounces (170mL) of olive oil**

- **One Tbsp of boiling water**

Place the egg yolks, salt, cayenne pepper, garlic and mustard in a bowl. Beat it with a wire whisk until it has thickened slightly. Beat in the oil slowly drop by drop, as you do with mayonnaise. Once you have used up all the oil, gradually beat in the boiling water. This is going to improve the consistency of this delicious mustard garlic butter.

I make this fresh every spring, especially when I have fresh herbs growing in my garden. I add one spring onion, all the green herbal leaves I can collect – including mint, parsley, thyme, marjoram, basil, – in small quantities to this garlic butter. Absolutely healthy and delicious. The family loves it, and the only problem is keeping up with their demands of a fresh stock, every 15 days.

That is because they need to slather everything, including chicken mayonnaise sandwiches, hot dogs, sausages, and anything else of which they can think with this garlic mustard butter.

You may ask why I do not use a blender to do the mixing. It somehow does not taste the same. Also, my particular blender does not have that cover attachment which allows the slow drop by drop oil mixing facility through a hole. So I improve my flabby arm muscle tone by beating by hand.

Gets out lots of accumulated anger and tension, especially when you are growling in your throat at the same time, and making other uncouth inarticulate noises! This adds interest to the proceedings!

Traditional Cooked Mustard Greens

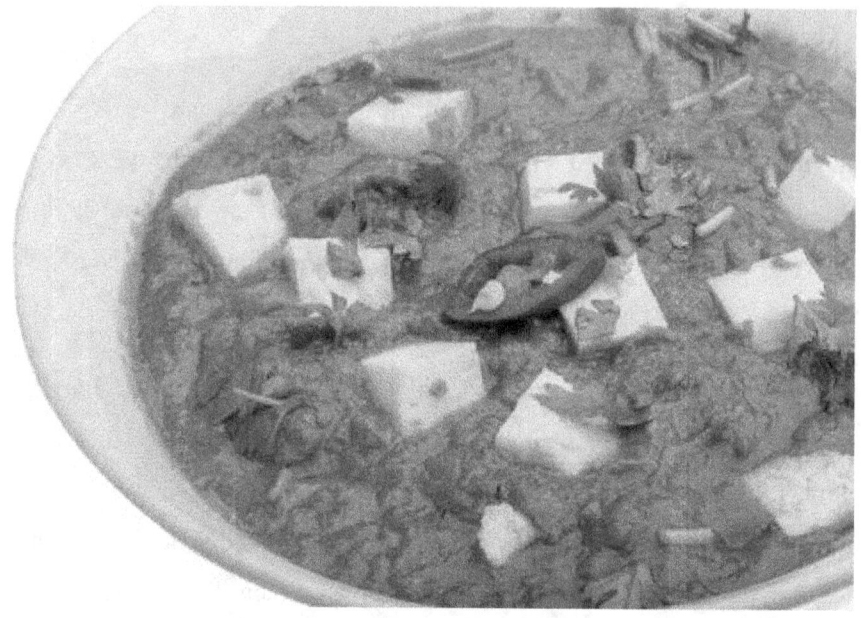

This has a lot of spinach and mustard plus fried cottage cheese chunks added to it.

Now this is something which is eaten every single day in the winter, in many parts of the Indian subcontinent. You can consider it to be the staple diet. No wonder one sleeps like a log in the afternoons after one has had traditional cooked mustard with dollops of homemade butter, and freshly churned buttermilk.

Cooked Mustard Greens

- 4 1/4 cups (1 kg) of mustard greens

- About 1/2 pound (250 g) of spinach

- Three to four cloves of crushed garlic

- 2 1/2 inch piece of ginger, chopped finely

- One green chopped chili

- Salt, to taste

- Two Tbsp of cornmeal

- 1 1/2 Tbsp of molasses/jaggery

As this is the traditional recipe, you will need to do the tempering with three tablespoons full of clarified butter, which is known as desi ghee. If you are health conscious, you may substitute butter instead of the concentrated clarified butter, but it somehow does not managed to taste the same. This tempering will also need one piece of ginger, finely chop, half a teaspoonful of red chili powder, and two green chillies finely chopped.

You are going to say, hey, where is the onion? Imagine Indian cuisine without onions? The onions are stuck on the prepared dish, to be eaten raw, along with Juliennes of ginger and full green chilies for all those who still like a bite with their mustard.

Wash and clean the mustard leaves, then remove the leaves and peel the stems. Start from the lower end and chop them finely. You are going to be the stems the way beans are strung. The addition of the stem to the spinach is going to make it tastier. The lower end is peeled, because it may not be so tender, but you can chop up the upper tender portion without doing any peeling.

Chop up the spinach leaves and mix with the mustard leaves.

A number of kids dislike spinach and mustard, because it is possible, they have not been introduced to this in the cooked form with its buttery consistency. This is definitely not going to be a soggy mess when it is dished up with hot bread.

Put the chopped greens with half a cup of water in a pan chop up the ginger, garlic and green chilli, very finely and add to the mixture. Add salt and start cooking on medium heat for 15 – 20 minutes. The leaves are going to "reduce" in size/quantity. Remove from the fire. Allow to cool.

Grind them to a coarse paste. Traditionally, this grinding is done in a pestle and mortar, but I use a blender. Do not grind too much and make it very smooth.

Add the corn flour to the mixture and allow to cook for another 15 minutes on low heat.

Tempering

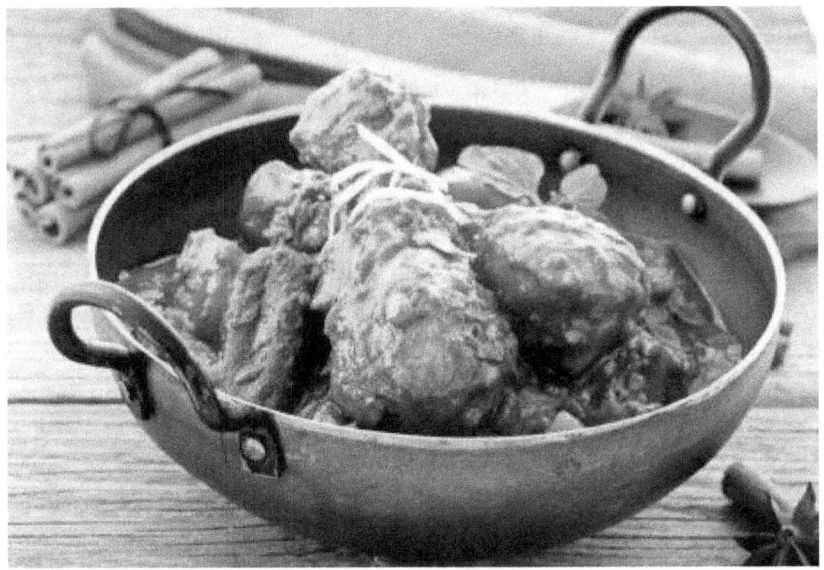

All that fat swimming on the gravy surface means this meat dish has been "tempered" with clarified butter. Greens can also be tempered after cooking.

For tempering, heat the clarified butter. Reduce the heat and add the green chillies and the ginger. Cook them until the ginger changes its color.

Remove the Wok from the fire and add red chilli powder. Now this is one procedure, which calls for open windows because your kitchen is going to be filled with the pungent aroma of tempering chilli powder. Add the clarified butter to the hot spinach, mix thoroughly and serve sizzling hot with fresh homemade butter, ginger strips, raw onion and green chillies.

In traditional Indian hotels, you may hear the sizzle of the tempering being done, followed with lots of smoke and eyes watering. This tempering is done right on the fire itself by the experienced cooks. They add the spinach to the boiling hot oil, which 9 times out of 10 catches fire with a swoosh and the onlookers saying appreciative aaaaaaahs![3] The cooks say that this is the last cooking stage. And their customers pay to see this final tempering, which is known as 'tadka.'

This tempering is also done to lentils(dal) and meat. Any excuse to eat Clarified butter with lots of dried spices and hot chillies!

Fresh mustard spinach should have tender leaves and tender stems.

---

[3] Well, as they say, somebody else is taking the risk and living dangerously is half the fun of eating traditional dishes. Otherwise, why would people want to eat Fugu or puffer fish, with its possibility of toxin poisoning?

Conclusion

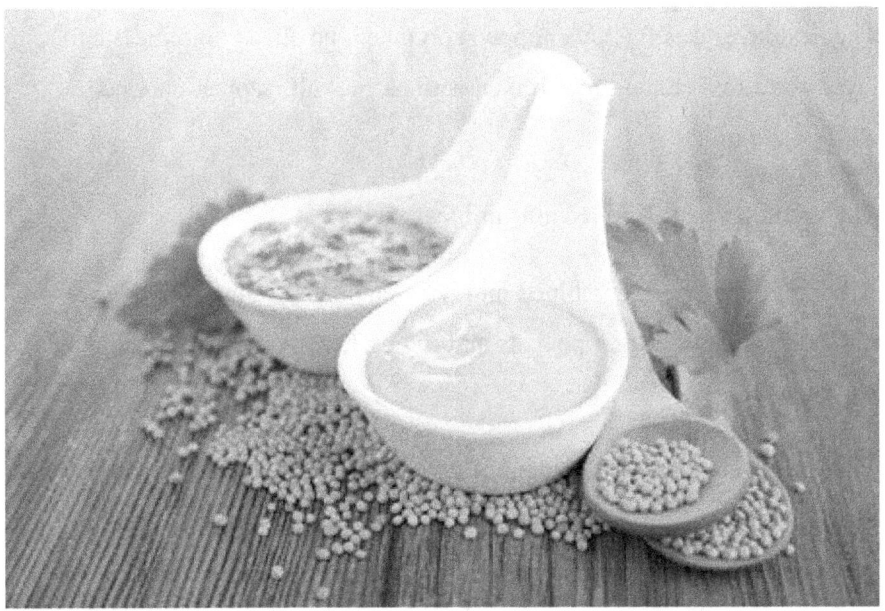

This book has introduced you to the magic of mustard. Mustard as a green eaten raw is delicious. It is even tastier when it is cooked.

Just last evening, I remember trying to analyze the ingredients in one of my favorite junk food burger/foot-long fillings –[4]

---

[4] I normally binge on junk food, once a month eating all sorts of burgers, hoagies, Subs, etc. in order to analyze what makes them so delicious and addictive to young and old, collectively. [Pathetic excuse, but hey, it works excellently to shut up my nagging conscience!]

Here was I with a mouthful of creamy meat filling which I could recognize as juicy boiled chicken, cooked in onions, ginger, garlic, tomatoes, spices, cream, and herbs.

The next layer was freshly chopped coriander and sliced onions. The third layer was a real cream sauce mixed with garlic, salt, pepper, chopped chillies and mint.

The fourth layer was boiled mustard leaves.

All of these had been combined into one delicious mishmash, hidden away into hollowed out Burger pockets and selling faster than hotcakes in that particular bakery.[5]

And I was paying the equivalent of dollar and five cents for this addictive burger -and a number of its brothers packed in a takeaway, to be eaten smothered in tomato ketchup and mustard at home, when I could make it equally easily at home.

And so I shall. I can always trim off the extra calories with swimming.

So remember, mustard, like Popeye's spinach may have got bad PR, down the ages, because of its pungency, but it is one of the most nutritious of greens known to man.

---

[5] The Baker always greets me with, "Ma'am, I was wondering why you took so long in coming here, I have not seen you this past month." He is always afraid that I might start making my own burgers, subs and foot- longs, after having stolen his recipe and stop buying them from him. And that is why each time he has an extra ingredient added to the burger. Last time it was sesame seeds, Nigella seeds and caraway seeds sprinkled on the burger. Aah, the list groweth...

Start growing your own greens now. Mustard can be grown indoors in containers. So now is the time to sow the seeds, and reap a bountiful harvest, before the summer comes in.

Live Long and Prosper!

Author Bio

Dueep Jyot Singh is a Management and IT Professional who managed to gather Postgraduate qualifications in Management and English and Degrees in Science, French and Education while pursuing different enjoyable career options like being an hospital administrator, IT,SEO and HRD Database Manager/ trainer, movie , radio and TV scriptwriter, theatre artiste and public speaker, lecturer in French, Marketing and Advertising, ex-Editor of Hearts On Fire (now known as Solstice) Books Missouri USA, advice columnist and cartoonist, publisher and Aviation School trainer, ex-moderator on Medico.in, banker, student councilor ,travelogue writer … among other things!

One fine morning, she decided that she had enough of killing herself by Degrees and went back to her first love -- writing. It's more enjoyable! She already has 48 published academic and 14 fiction- in- different- genre books under her belt.

When she is not designing websites or making Graphic design illustrations for clients , she is browsing through old bookshops hunting for treasures, of which she has an enviable collection – including R.L. Stevenson, O.Henry, Dornford Yates, Maurice Walsh, De Maupassant, Victor Hugo, Sapper, C.N. Williamson, "Bartimeus" and the crown of her collection- Dickens "The Old Curiosity Shop," and "Martin Chuzzlewit" and so on… Just call her "Renaissance Woman") - collecting herbal remedies, acting like Universal Helping Hand/Agony Aunt, or escaping to her dear mountains for a bit of exploring, collecting herbs and plants and trekking.

Check out some of the other JD-Biz Publishing books

Gardening Series on Amazon

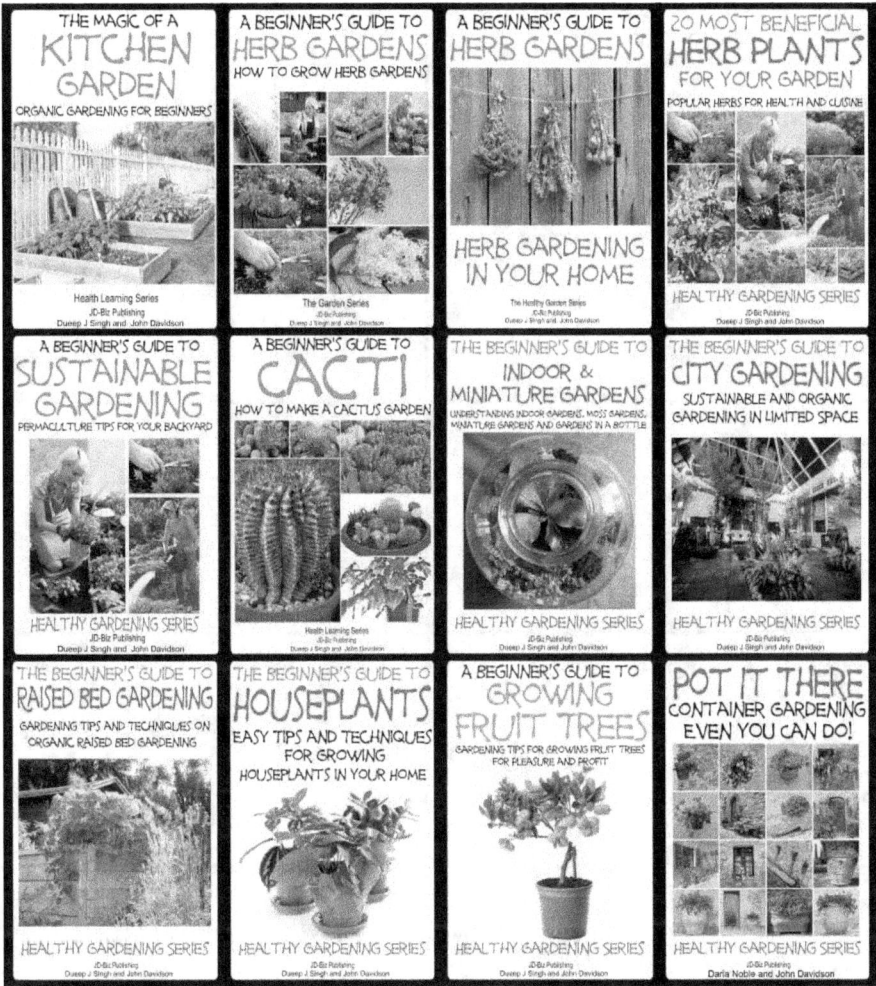

Health Learning Series

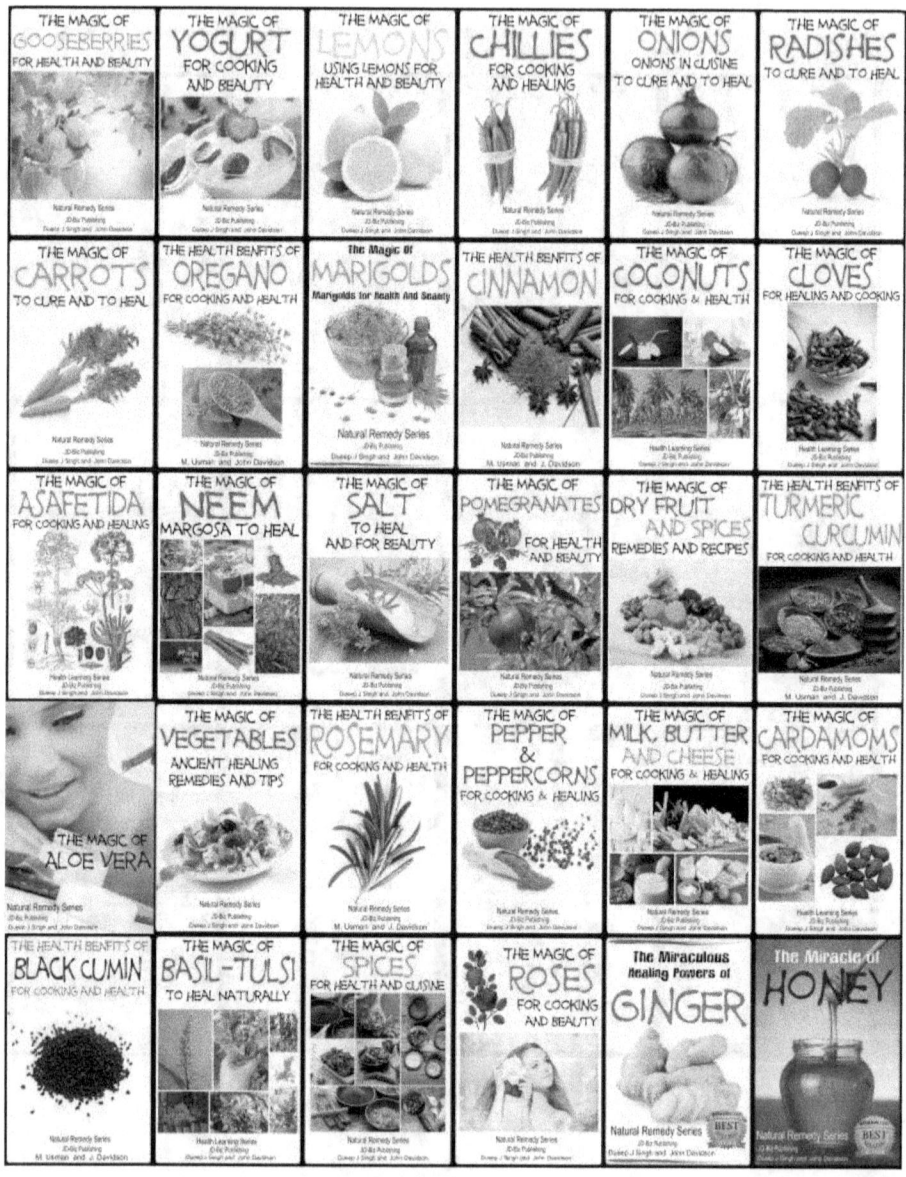

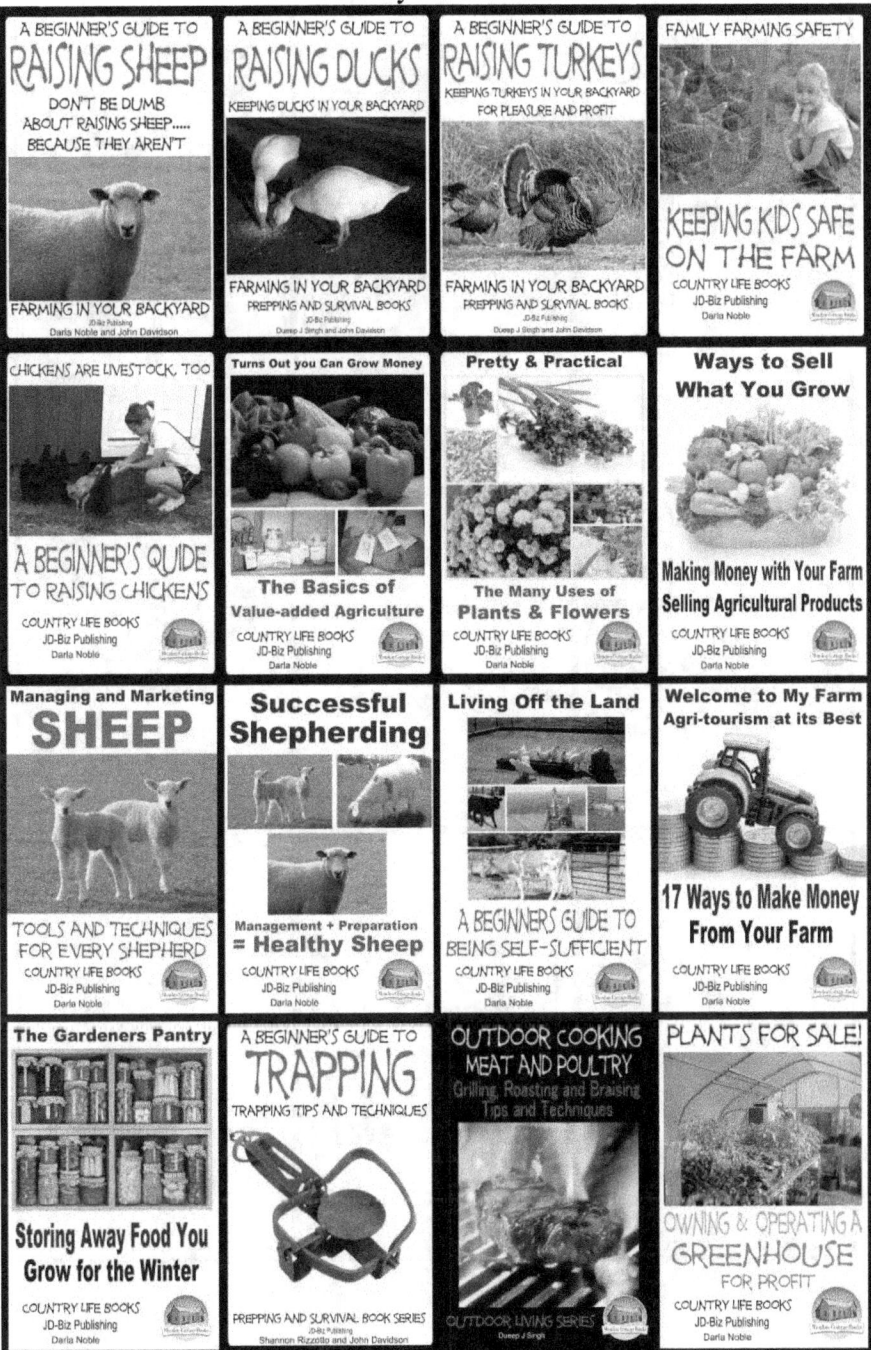

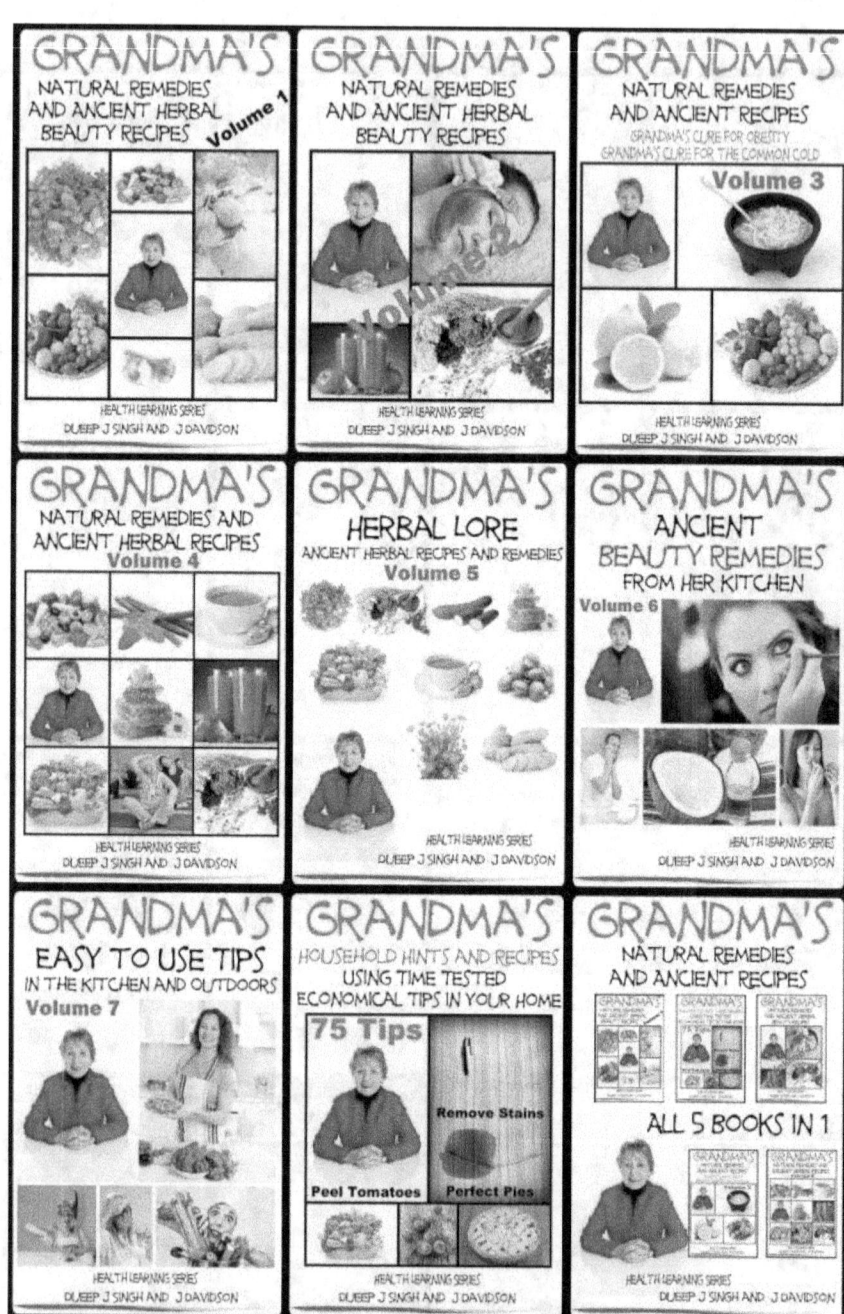

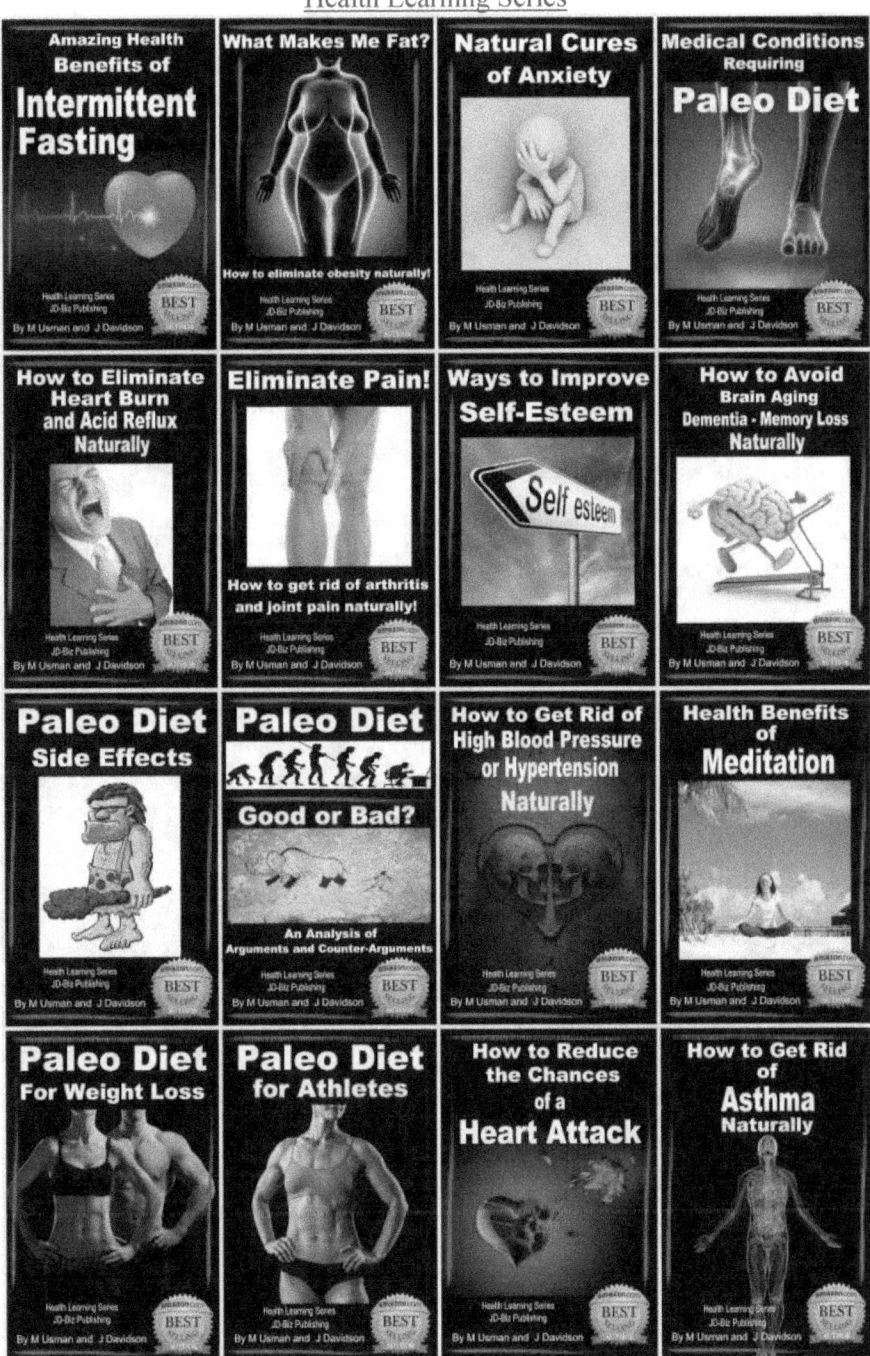

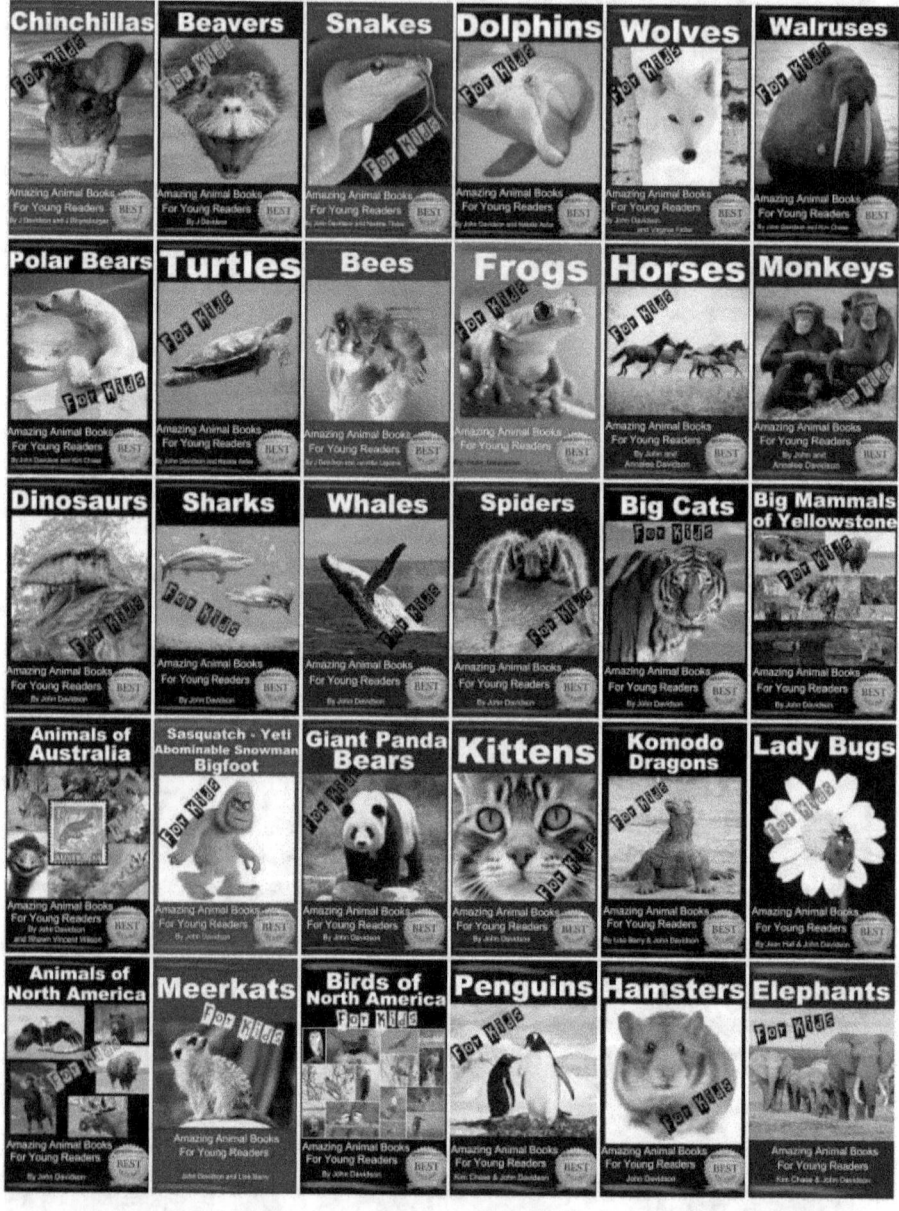

Learn To Draw Series

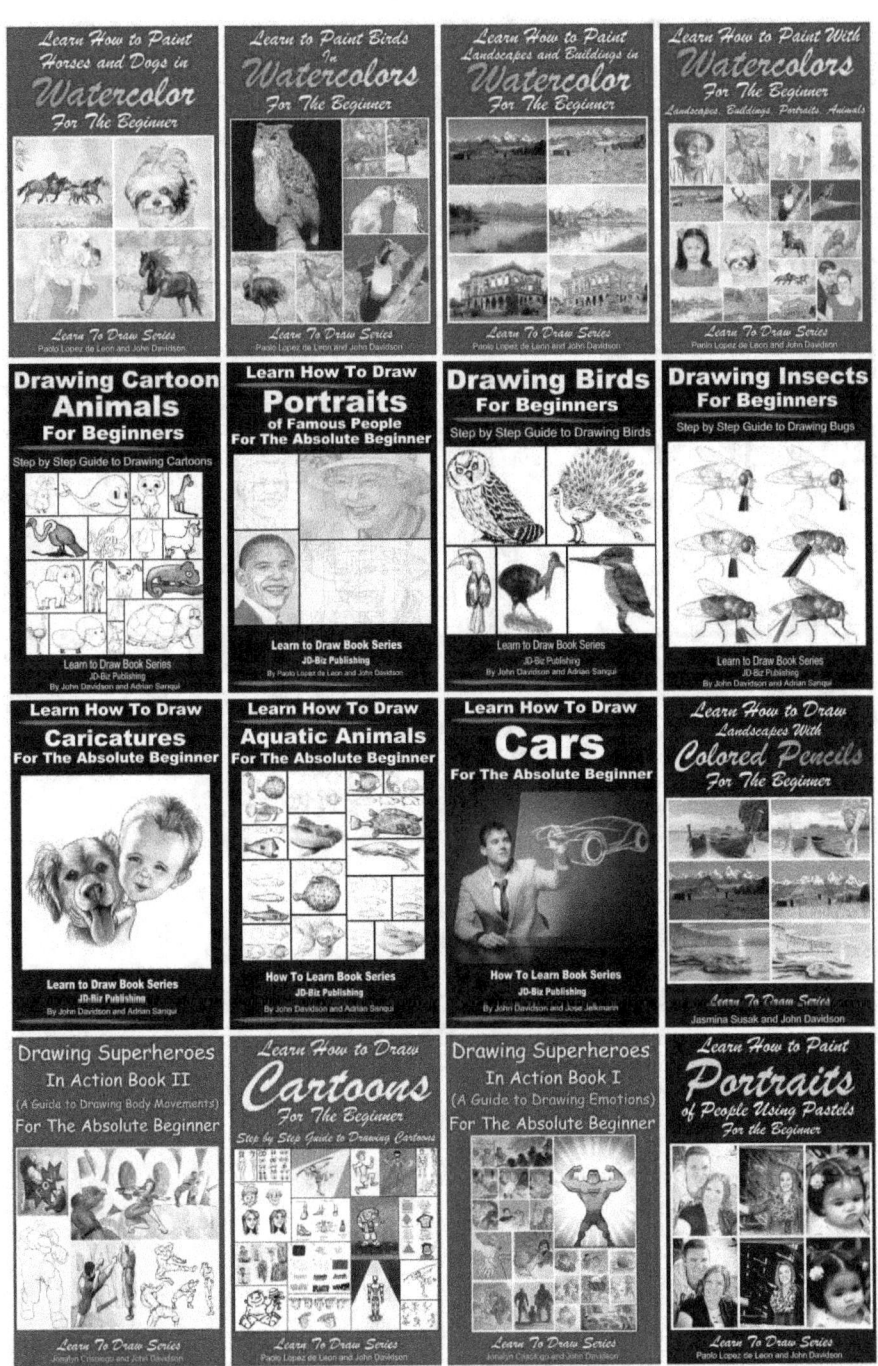

How to Build and Plan Books

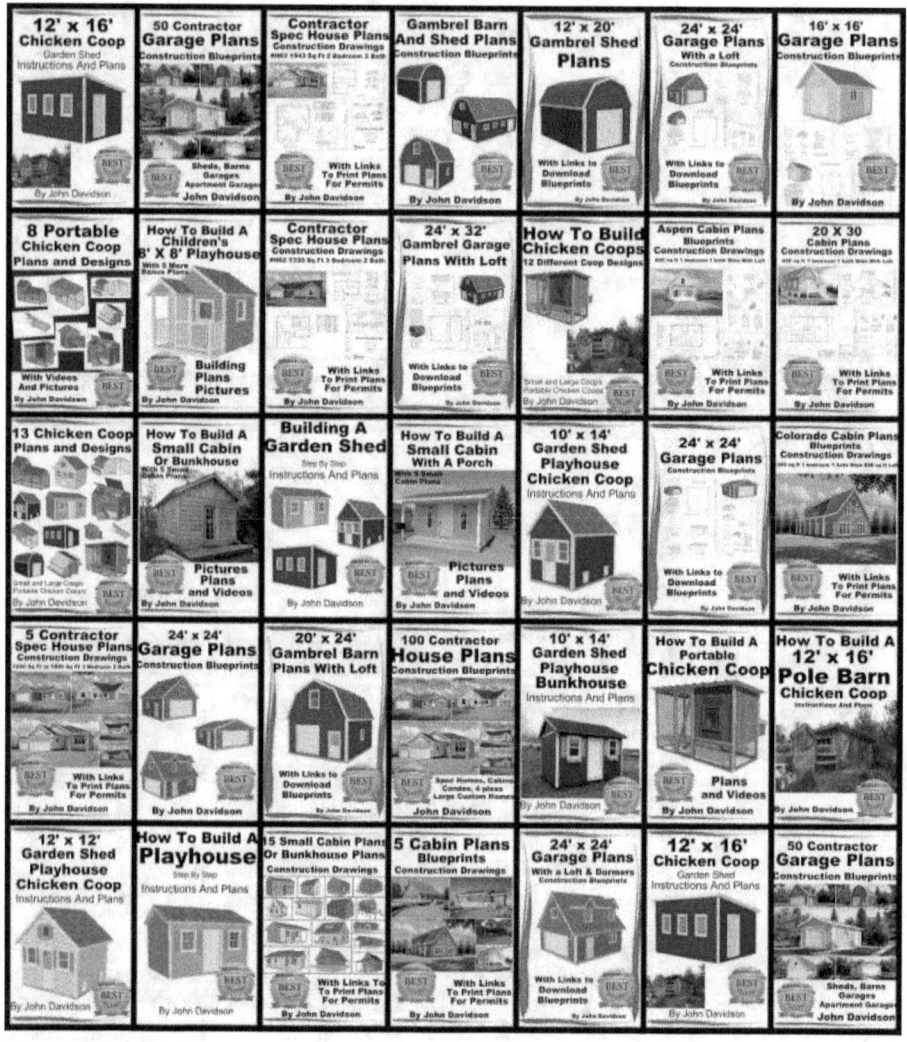

Entrepreneur Book Series

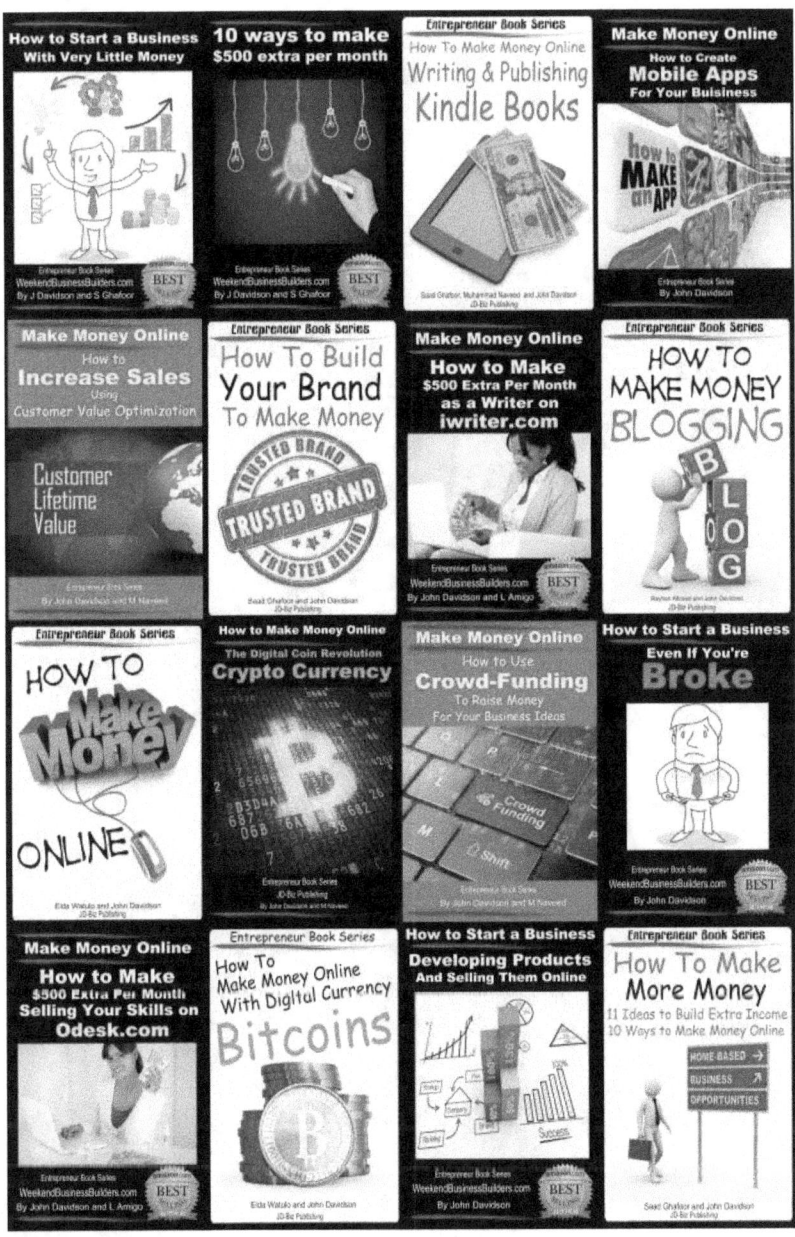

Our books are available at

1. Amazon.com

2. Barnes and Noble

3. Itunes

4. Kobo

5. Smashwords

6. Google Play Books

Publisher

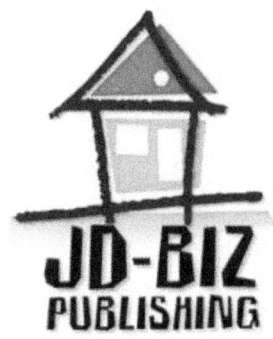

JD-Biz Corp

P O Box 374

Mendon, Utah 84325

http://www.jd-biz.com/

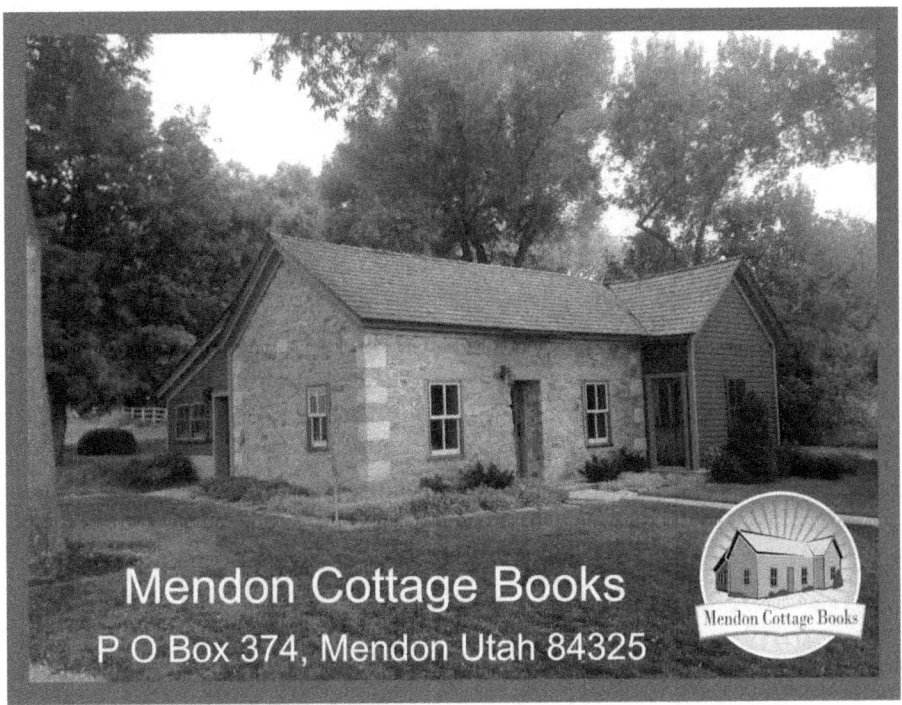

Mendon Cottage Books

P O Box 374, Mendon Utah 84325